Contents

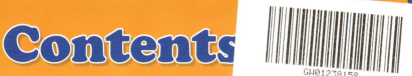

	Pages
You're Pregnant!	4-5
Your Baby in the Womb	6-9
Healthy Eating	10-11
Drinking during Pregnancy	12-13
Smoking during Pregnancy	14-15
Sex in Pregnancy	16-17
Getting Prepared	18-19
Birth & Labour Stage 1	20-21
Pain Relief in Labour	22-23
Birth and Labour Stages 2+3	24-25
Breastfeeding/Bathing	26-27
After the Birth/Contraception	28-29
Support	30-31

You're Pregnant!

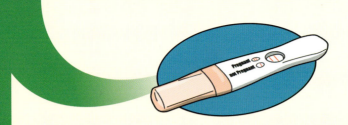

Congratulations!

Have you booked with your midwife? If not your midwife can be contacted via your GP's surgery *(there's no need to see your GP)*.

Telling the father

Telling the father is very important; he is equally as responsible as you are. Do not put this off as the longer it takes the harder it will be.

Girls often say, 'If I get pregnant he will finish with me.' Well if he does he wasn't worth keeping!

Remember this will be a big shock to him and he may need space for a few days to think. The time to think alone may do you both good as you may see things more clearly.

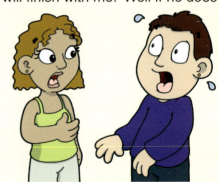

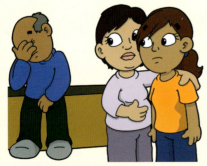

Telling your parents

You may be scared of telling your parents, many people say, 'If I told my mum and dad I was pregnant they would kick me out.' But more often than not they come round and support you. They will be shocked but, you are their child and they want what's best for you.

'My parents were upset at first, and then they were okay about it.'
Kirsty aged 18, mum to 16 month old son

Your Rights

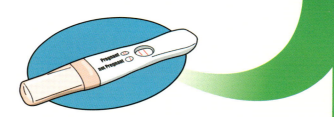

As a pregnant woman you are entitled to 52 weeks maternity leave, regardless of how long you have worked for an employer, how old you are or how many hours you do, providing that you give 15 weeks notice before your baby is due.

If you are at school or college you have the same rights as pregnant staff - you cannot be told to leave just because you are pregnant.

You will be able to claim some of the following allowances depending upon your circumstances:

- Sure Start Maternity Grant
- Child Benefit
- Healthy Start Scheme
- Housing Benefit
- Statutory Maternity Pay (SMP)
- Maternity Allowance (MA)
- Universal Credit

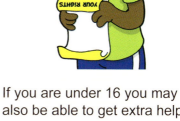

If you are under 16 you may also be able to get extra help from Social Services.

For FREE advice on exactly what you are entitled to contact your local Citizens Advice Bureau (CAB) or log on to www.citizensadvice.org.uk and follow the Adviceguide from the home page.

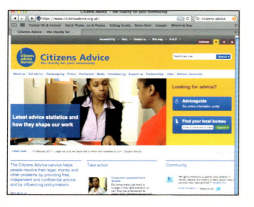

Your Baby in the Womb

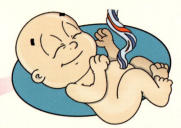

Before 4 weeks the egg is moving along the fallopian tube and becomes implanted in the womb.

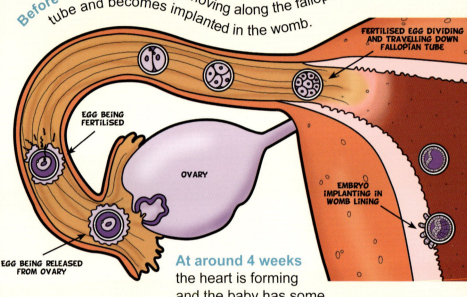

At around 4 weeks the heart is forming and the baby has some of its own blood vessels, which are linked to you. These will become the umbilical cord.

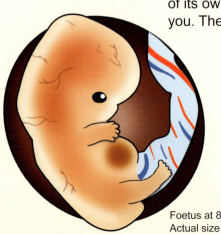

At 6 - 8 weeks there is a bump where the heart is and it can be seen beating on an ultrasound scan. The brain can be seen as a bump in the head as it is developing.

Foetus at 8 weeks
Actual size = 8 - 10mm

Your Baby in the Womb

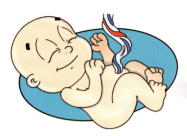

At 9 - 12 weeks the face has started forming slowly and the baby now has a mouth and a tongue. The heart, lungs, liver and kidneys have begun to develop.

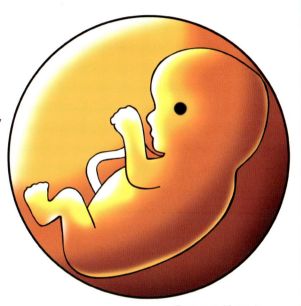

Foetus at 10 weeks
Size = about 22mm

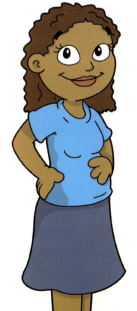

By weeks 13 - 15 the foetus is fully formed. It has organs, muscles and bones. The baby's sex organs have now developed. This is the period when most women begin to show the pregnancy.

The size of the foetus is about 85mm

Your Baby in the Womb

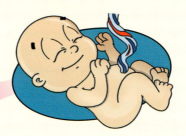

During weeks 16 - 24 the baby's eyelashes, eyebrows and fingerprints are beginning to form and the baby is growing quite quickly. Usually at this time you will have an ultrasound scan to check that everything is okay with the baby. You may also start to feel the baby's movements.

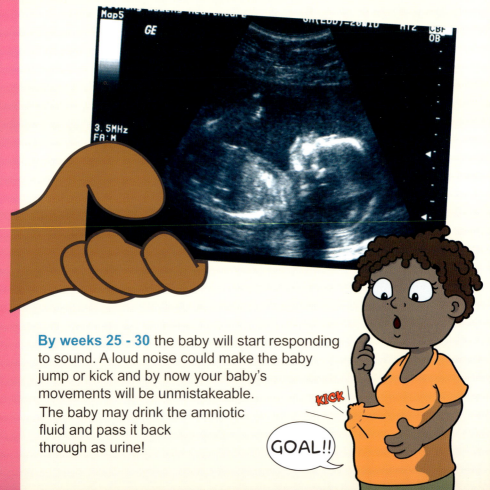

By weeks 25 - 30 the baby will start responding to sound. A loud noise could make the baby jump or kick and by now your baby's movements will be unmistakeable.
The baby may drink the amniotic fluid and pass it back through as urine!

Your Baby in the Womb

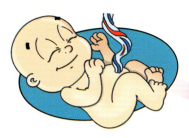

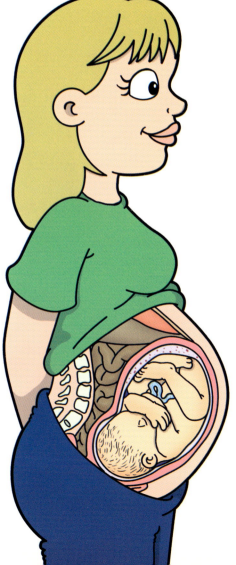

Maternity Clothes

Most high street fashion shops have great maternity ranges, so you don't need to squeeze into clothes that are too small!

If you are struggling to finance maternity clothes you may be able to get help from the Social Fund. Contact your local Citizens Advice Bureau for details.

In weeks 31 - 40 the baby is growing and preparing for birth. You may see your baby kicking and moving around inside you.

By about 32 weeks the baby's head is moving down ready to engage into your pelvis, although sometimes the baby's head does not engage until labour has started.

Healthy Eating

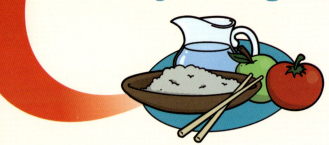

Healthy eating is really important now, as you have to provide nutrients for your baby as well as yourself. There are some foods which you will have to avoid during your pregnancy so speak to your midwife for more information.

To keep healthy during pregnancy every day you will need to eat:

- Plenty of bread, pasta, rice or potatoes - try the wholegrain versions as these contain lots of fibre and can help you stop feeling constipated.

- Five portions of fruit and vegetables - these can be fresh, frozen, tinned, dried or a glass of fruit juice to provide vital vitamins, minerals and fibre.

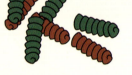

- Three portions of dairy foods such as milk, cheese, yoghurts - these contain calcium and protein which helps to keep your bones strong and are vital for the healthy growth of your baby's bones.

- Two servings of lean meat, chicken or fish. If you are a vegetarian you will need to take protein from pulses, nuts, milk (including soya milk), eggs and cheese.

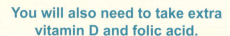

You will also need to take extra vitamin D and folic acid.

You may be able to get Healthy Start Vouchers to help pay for some of these foods and vitamins. See your midwife for details.

Cravings

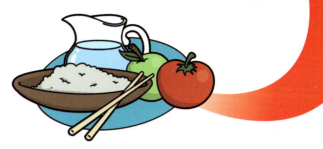

Cravings, the urge to eat certain things that you wouldn't normally eat, can often happen during pregnancy. It's quite normal!

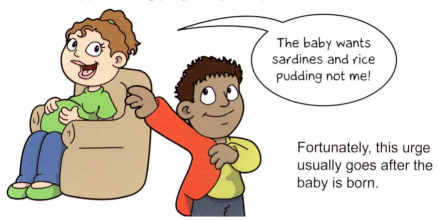

The baby wants sardines and rice pudding not me!

Fortunately, this urge usually goes after the baby is born.

Putting on Weight

During pregnancy some women's appetites increase and they need to eat more than they did before. This is fine as long as you stick to healthy foods.

Try replacing:

- Crisps with low fat crackers
- Tea/coffee with fruit juices or water
- White bread with wholemeal bread

Remember: You are NOT eating for two!

If you are feeling unwell or sick during your pregnancy and are unable to eat anything, see your midwife as soon as possible for help and advice.

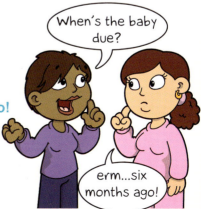

When's the baby due?

erm...six months ago!

Drinking During Pregnancy

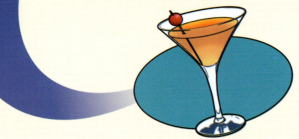

For many years, researchers thought that it was not harmful to drink alcohol occasionally during pregnancy, but the latest research has shown that even occasional drinking can be harmful to your unborn child.

- **Drinking during pregnancy is linked to:**

  - Miscarriage
  - Stillbirth
  - Brain damage to your baby

  Heavy or frequent drinking can seriously damage your baby's health.

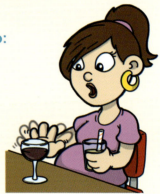

No one can make you stop drinking, but can only advise against it.

A guide to the number of units of alcohol contained in drinks:

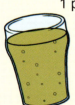

1 pint of 4% lager, beer or cider
=
2.3 units

1 bottle (275ml) of 5% alcopop
=
1.4 units

a single measure of spirits
=
1 unit

a standard glass of wine
=
1.75 units

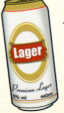

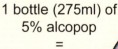

1 can (440ml) of 5% lager
=
2.2 units

Drinking During Pregnancy

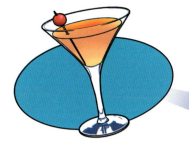

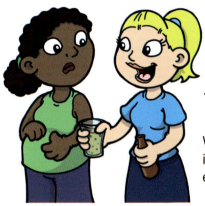

Well I don't see how a couple will hurt...go on!

When you are socialising you may find it difficult to avoid the urge to drink, especially if friends are encouraging you.

Hints to avoiding the urge to drink whilst socialising:

- Drink a non-alcoholic drink that you enjoy.
- Drink juice in a spirit glass with a mixer stick, as this may stop people asking you why you are not drinking.
- Try non-alcoholic lager.

If you are finding not drinking alcohol a problem, you can talk to your doctor/midwife or you can contact the **Alcohol Helpline** on:

FREE PHONE 0800 917 8282
(24 hours a day, 7 days a week)

Illegal drugs are extremely harmful to both you and your baby. If you need help to stop using drugs see your GP or midwife.

Some medicines can also harm your baby and should not be taken without medical advice.

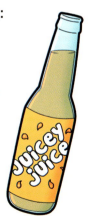

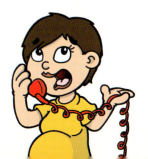

Smoking During Pregnancy

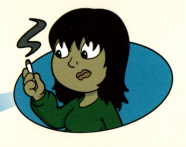

Smoking passes carbon monoxide to your lungs reducing the oxygen to your bloodstream, which during pregnancy means less oxygen is getting to your baby. The nicotine can also make your baby's heart beat faster.

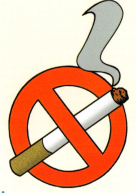

Smoking during pregnancy is linked to:

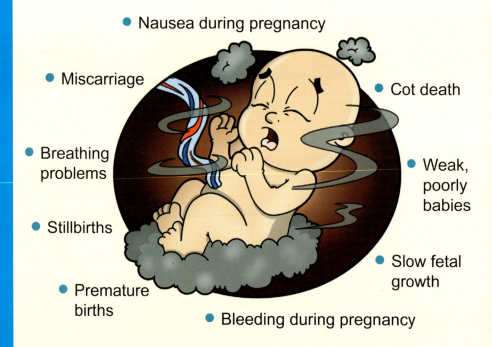

- Nausea during pregnancy
- Miscarriage
- Cot death
- Breathing problems
- Weak, poorly babies
- Stillbirths
- Slow fetal growth
- Premature births
- Bleeding during pregnancy

Smoking poses a serious health risk, not only to you, but also to your baby as well!

Smoking During Pregnancy

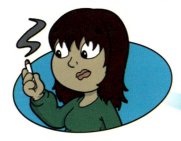

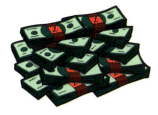

A good way to motivate yourself whilst giving up smoking is to think of all the money you could save - money that could come in handy once the baby arrives.

No. of cigarettes a day	5	10	20	40
Daily Cost	£1.63	£3.25	£6.50	£13.00
Weekly Cost	£11.38	£22.75	£45.50	£91.00
Monthly Cost	£45.50	£91.00	£182.00	£364.00
Yearly Cost	£593.13	£1186.25	£2372.50	£4745.00

These figures are calculated on an average packet of 20 cigarettes costing £6.50

Quitting smoking isn't easy but it's do-able and there is so much help out there to make it easier.

If you are finding giving up smoking a problem, you can talk to your doctor/midwife or you can contact the **NHS Pregnancy Smoking Helpline** on:

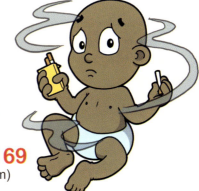

FREE PHONE 0800 169 9169
(Mon - Fri, 9am - 8pm   Sat - Sun, 11am - 5pm)

You have the CHOICE not to smoke, and so should your baby!

Sex in Pregnancy

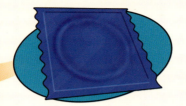

Sex is an important part of a relationship.

The good news is that it is perfectly safe to have sex when you are pregnant.

However, once your waters have broken, you should not have sex as there is nothing protecting your baby and it is prone to infection.

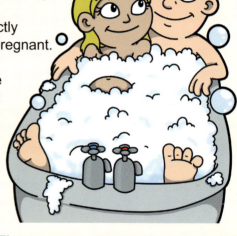

Beware of STIs

Sexually Transmitted Infections (STIs) can be very harmful to your unborn child. It is now even more important to make sure that you and your partner do not have a STI.

Visit your GP or CASH (*Contraceptive and Sexual Health*) Service for a check up. Your results can even be sent via confidential text to your mobile phone.

The number of my local CASH Service

Sex in Pregnancy

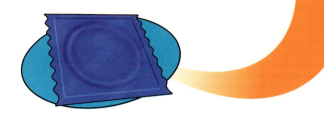

It's important for you and your partner to try and stay strong as a couple. The first few months of parenting will strain your relationship, so it's important to stand together as a team and share things. Continuing an active sex life during pregnancy may help your relationship stay relatively normal.

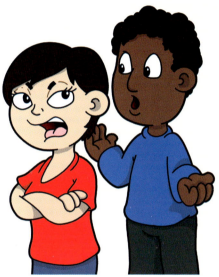

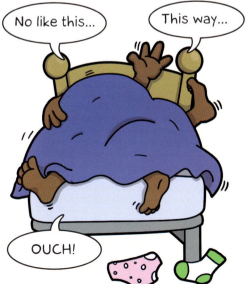

You can have fun experimenting with different positions to find the most comfortable position for you both.

Most women find it more comfortable to be on top because of the baby bump and sore breasts.

17

Getting Prepared

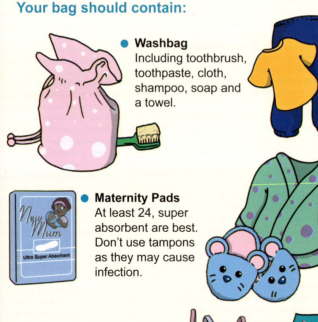

In the last few weeks of pregnancy you will need to get prepared for hospital, the baby and coming home.

This period can be very exciting, or it can be quite scary for some people. You will need to pack all the final items for your hospital stay by 36 weeks, just in case you go into premature labour.

Your bag should contain:

- **Washbag**
Including toothbrush, toothpaste, cloth, shampoo, soap and a towel.

- **Clothes**
Lots of people will visit and you may not feel comfortable in your PJs. You will also need clothes for coming home.

- **Night Clothes**
4 nighties or PJs, a dressing gown and slippers. The average hospital stay is 1-2 nights.

- **Maternity Pads**
At least 24, super absorbent are best. Don't use tampons as they may cause infection.

- **Knickers**
At least 6 pairs of old knickers or disposable paper pants. It's nice to change often as it's like a very heavy period.

- **2-3 Nursing Bras (if breastfeeding)**
Remember breasts will be bigger than usual and may be sore.

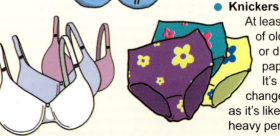

Getting Prepared

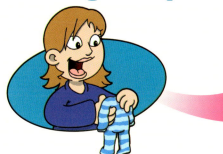

You will also need to pack things for the baby.
This is something that you will need to do everytime you leave the house from now on! The best thing to think when you don't know what to pack is **pack everything!**

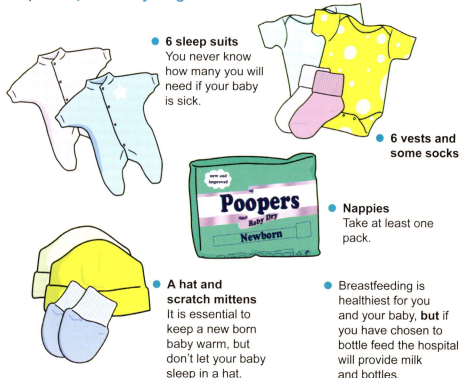

- **6 sleep suits**
  You never know how many you will need if your baby is sick.

- **6 vests and some socks**

- **Nappies**
  Take at least one pack.

- **A hat and scratch mittens**
  It is essential to keep a new born baby warm, but don't let your baby sleep in a hat.

- **Breastfeeding is healthiest for you and your baby, but** if you have chosen to bottle feed the hospital will provide milk and bottles.

Your feelings and emotions may suddenly change before the birth and you may start to feel the urge to clean everything and get the baby's room ready for his/her arrival. This is known as nesting and may last until the baby is born, it doesn't always happen, but it's completely normal.

Birth & Labour

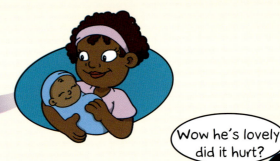

The Birth

Finally after nearly 40 weeks you will be wanting to give birth to your baby, even if it's just wanting to get it over and done with!

People have different expectations of labour. Some think the worst whilst others think it will be easy.

If you're terrified about labour don't be! Millions of women have done it before you and millions will do it after you. Some people even go on to have another child, so it can't be that bad!

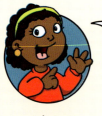

"My best bit of pregnancy was the birth."

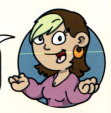

"Stretch marks and sickness were the worst."

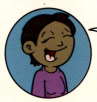

"Tiredness was the biggest problem for me."

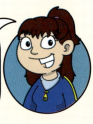

"When the baby kicked and I realised I was a mum, that was the best."

When asked, 'What was the best and worst thing about pregnancy?' only 2 out of 30 young mums said labour was the worst part!

Birth & Labour

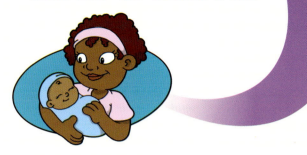

Labour is split into three stages:

Stage One: Dilation of the cervix

No one can tell you when labour will start, less than 5% of babies arrive on their due date. The signs of labour starting can be:

- Back ache
- The waters breaking
- Contractions

- Nausea & vomiting
- Diarrhoea
- A show - this is the mucus plug which seals the cervix until labour

If you are having any of these signs, ring the labour ward immediately. The most common sign of labour starting is contractions. This is when the abdomen tightens and relaxes. The closer to the birth you get the stronger the pain will become.

Contractions shrink the uterus which gradually opens the cervix to 10cm - known as fully dilated. Towards the end of the contractions you may feel the urge to push.

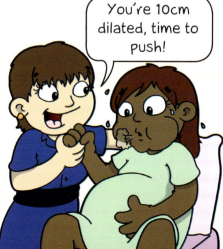

You're 10cm dilated, time to push!

Pain Relief in Labour

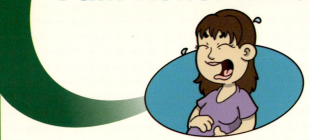

Antenatal classes are a great way to learn about labour, the different types of pain relief that are available and how to cope without pain relief. You can ask about:

Natural methods

- Breathing exercises
- Massage
- Homeopathy
- Aromatherapy
- Birth Hypnosis
- Water Birth
- Reflexology
- Acupuncture

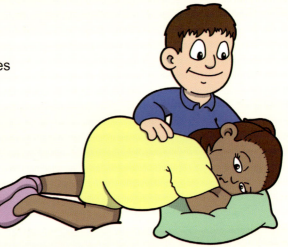

Gas and Air

- 50% laughing gas and 50% oxygen.
- You give it to yourself.
- It has no ill effect on you or your baby.
- It only takes 15 - 20 seconds to work.
- It can make you feel a bit drunk.

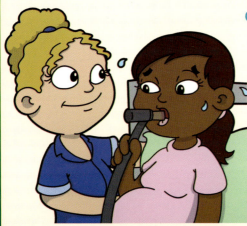

Pain Relief in Labour

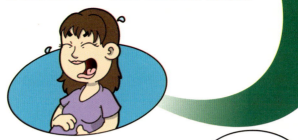

Pethidine

- Powerful sedative that calms you down and may make you go to sleep.
- The midwife will inject it into your leg.
- It takes about 20 minutes to work and lasts for 2 - 4 hours.
- It crosses the placenta which may make the baby sleepy and cause problems with breathing and feeding.

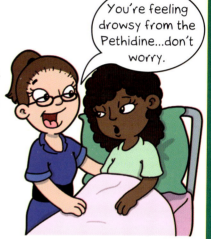

Epidural

- A continous, powerful dose of painkillers injected into your spine.
- The doctor passes a thin plastic tube into your back.
- Most women have an almost pain free labour.
- Slightly more likely to have complications in labour such as ventouse or forceps deliveries or a Caesarean section.

Talk to your midwife

Midwives don't withhold pain relief but there are certain times for certain drugs, you should discuss beforehand the type of pain relief you feel comfortable with.

Birth & Labour

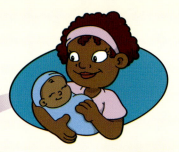

Stage Two: The baby's birth

In this stage it is better if you move around to find a position that suits you and eases the pain a little. Once you feel the urge to push, and the midwife has checked that you are ready, you can start to push with every contraction.

With a contraction you push into your bottom like you are having a poo. In between contractions you will need to rest and keep energy for the next push.

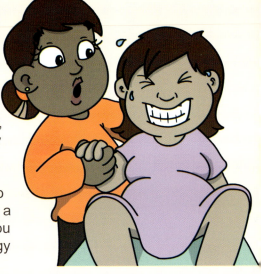

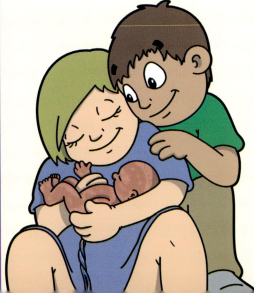

When the baby's head can be seen the midwife will tell you to push gently. After the baby's head has been born, one more push and the body should follow soon after.

This is the hardest stage of labour, but it's worth it. The pain doesn't matter once your baby is born. It is the most magical experience of your life.

Birth & Labour

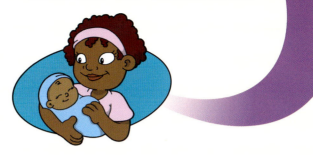

Stage Three: Delivery of the placenta

If you have had a normal birth the placenta can be delivered naturally which usually takes about an hour. Alternatively the midwife can give you an injection of a synthetic hormone which should speed it up to about 5 minutes. The injection is given in your leg as the baby is being born, it may also help the womb to contract and stop heavy bleeding once the placenta is out.

Afterwards

- You will be offered skin to skin contact with your baby as soon as possible after the birth. This helps to calm your baby. It is good for all babies and also helps to get breastfeeding off to a good start. During this time you and your partner can spend time together and get to meet your baby properly.

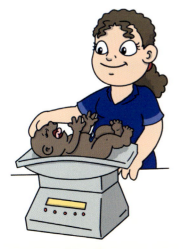

- After your baby has had it's first feed you will be given stitches if you have had a deep tear or cut.

- Your baby will be examined, weighed and given 2 bands with your name on.

- The midwife will help you to wash and freshen up.

Breastfeeding

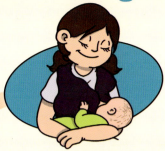

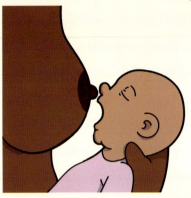

- Breast milk contains everything your baby needs and will change as your baby grows.

- Make sure you get your copy of 'Off to the best start' breastfeeding leaflet.

- From birth you should breastfeed your baby as often and for as long as your baby wants.

- The key to succesful breastfeeding is positioning and attaching your baby.

- Breastfeeding shouldn't hurt. If it does ask your midwife for help.

- Breastfeed for at least six months.

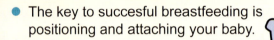
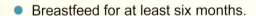
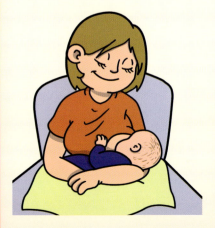

You can breastfeed when you're out and about without other people knowing - it just takes a little practice.

If you want someone else to feed your baby you can express some of your milk once your breastfeeding has become established.

Bathing

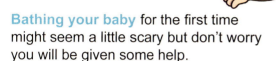

Bathing your baby for the first time might seem a little scary but don't worry you will be given some help.

You don't need any lotions or potions just plain water.

Don't wash baby's eyes unless they become infected. Then wash with cool boiled water.

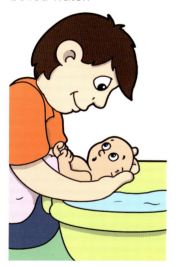

You don't need to bath your baby every day, but you should wash your baby's face, neck, hands and bottom carefully each day.

Give yourself some time when learning to bath your baby. You'll be nervous at first, but you are the expert on your baby.

You also need to clean your baby's bottom carefully each time you change a nappy to prevent soreness.

Change nappies on the floor or keep everything close by and don't leave baby for a second.

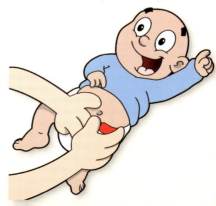

After the Birth

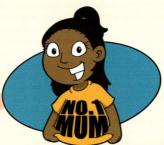

With the strain of the birth and caring for your baby, it may take a while until you are ready to resume your sex life!

When you choose to have sex again it is for you and your partner to discuss, **however** you should wait for at least a few weeks after the birth to give your body time to heal completely.

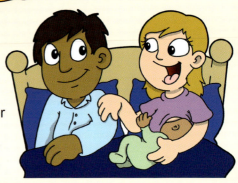

If you feel a little tightness, dryness or discomfort during sex, especially if you have had stitches, lubrication can help.

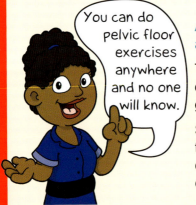

You can do pelvic floor exercises anywhere and no one will know.

Ask your midwife or health visitor about EXERCISES

The muscles holding your womb may loosen during childbirth and exercises can help you get these get back into shape.

Some women find after they have given birth that they may wee a little bit when they laugh or even run for the bus! 'Pelvic Floor' exercises will help to stop this happening.

Periods

- If you breastfeed your periods may not return until after you stop feeding.
- If you decide not to breastfeed your periods can return as early as 5-8 weeks after the birth of your baby.
- You can get pregnant again BEFORE you have a period.

Contraception

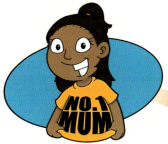

Contraception

Probably the last thing you will be thinking about is contraception. **But don't get caught out!**

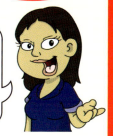

A lot of unplanned pregnancies happen in the first few months after childbirth.

Talk to your midwife, GP or family planning nurse to find out more about the different methods of contraception to use after the birth and decide the best one for you.

Some things to consider:

- ALL forms of contraception will protect you from unplanned pregnancies but condoms will also protect you from STIs.

- A contraceptive injection or implant cannot be given until 21-28 days after the birth.

- The coil (IUD) can be fitted after 4 weeks when your uterus has returned to its normal shape and size.

- Breastfeeding mums still need contraception, but should not use the combined pill.

- The Emergency Contraceptive Pill should not be used as a regular form of contraception. It can be taken up to 72 hours after unprotected sex, but the earlier it is taken the more effective it is.

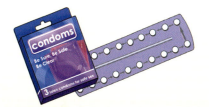

Don't forget that contraception is FREE and easily available from your GP, health professional or family planning clinic.

Support

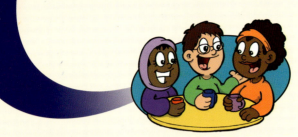

All parents and parents-to-be need support from other people.

Your support network may include:
- Family
- Friends
- Neighbours
- Midwife/ Health Visitor
- Doctors
- Teachers
- Community Leaders

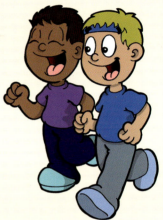

Family, friends and neighbours can be a great source of informal advice, providing a listening ear, hands on practical help and of course babysitting.

Your midwife, health visitor, or doctor will always be there to provide professional advice and support, and can also introduce you to other support networks in your area.

Try these great places to meet other parents:
- Antenatal Classes
- Children's Centres
- Parenting Groups
- Toddler Groups
- Single Parent Groups

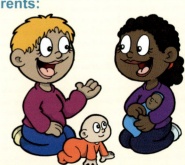

Remember, it is important to make time for you.
If you are tired and stressed both you and your baby will suffer.